About the Book

In-toeing, out-toeing, flatfeet, knock-knees, bowlegs, toe-walking, sudden refusal to walk: these afflictions of childhood are so common that together, they affect *all* children at some time during their growth and development.

Controversy abounds regarding the causes and cure of these problems. Pediatricians, orthopedic surgeons, podiatrists, grandmothers, and shoe salesmen all have strong opinions, yet all so conflicting! For any one of these problems, advice ranges from doing nothing, to wearing shoes, to wearing braces, and even to having surgery! The myths surrounding these conditions even cause professionals to be confused. What is a parent to do?

This book, written by a Harvard trained pediatric orthopedic surgeon, is an attempt to set the record straight. Writing in simple conversational style, he draws on experience and documented research findings to distinguish for the reader fact from fiction; he answers questions all parents have about their children's feet and leg problems. An especially useful chapter on shoes describes how parents should select shoes for their young ones.

Packed with practical information and advice, this book is a reading *must* for all who care about children's feet, whether parent or professional, but especially parents.

About the Author

Andrew K. C. Chong, M.D., is an orthopedic surgeon in private practice in Wheaton, Illinois. His interest in children's feet and leg problems led him to a clinical fellowship at Children's Hospital Medical Center in Boston (of Harvard University) where he did clinical research on children's gait and feet problems. He has published several papers in professional journals, as well as contributed to scientific meetings on children's feet and gait problems.

He is a Fellow of the Royal College of Surgeons of Edinburgh (U.K.), Royal College of Surgeons of Canada, and the American College of Surgeons.

In addition to his active practice, Dr. Chong is an orthopedic consultant for the Division of Services for Crippled Children, University of Illinois, and the Muscular Dystrophy Association of America.

IS YOUR CHILD WALKING RIGHT?

Parents' Guide to Little Feet

by
Andrew K. C. Chong, M.D.

Illustrations by
James S. Craig

Wheaton Resource Corp.
P.O. Box 1149
Wheaton, IL. 60189

Wheaton Resource Corporation, Box 1149, Wheaton, Illinois 60189

IS YOUR CHILD WALKING RIGHT?

Cover design by Joe Ragont
Cover photo by Jim Steere
Internal illustrations by James Craig

Distribution to the book trade by Chicago Review Press, 814 N. Franklin, Chicago, IL 60610

NOTICE: This book is not intended as a substitute for the medical advice of physicians. The reader should consult a physician in matters relating to his or her child's health and particularly in regards to any symptoms which may require diagnosis or medical attention. Neither the author nor the publisher shall be responsible for any harm or injury resulting from interpretations of the materials in this book.

First printing, 1986. Second printing, 1988. Third printing, 1990. Fourth printing, 1991.
Printed in the United States of America
96 95 94 93 92 91   9 8 7 6 5 4

Library of Congress Cataloging in Publication Data

Chong, Andrew K. C., M.D.
  Is Your Child Walking Right?

  1. Chong, Andrew K. C., M.D.   2. Children—Foot and leg.   3. Health—walking problems in children.
  85-052171
  ISBN: 0-936657-00-6

Acknowledgments

So many people have given of their time and expertise in the writing of this book that I hesitate to mention names lest I miss even one. But I would be remiss if I fail to mention the following.

Dr. Mervin Letts, M.D., Professor of Orthopedics at the University of Manitoba and Dr. Robert Rosenthal, M.D., Assistant Clinical Professor of Orthopedics at Harvard Medical School, and Dr. John E. Hall M.D., Professor of Orthopedics at Harvard Medical School, my teachers;

Dr. William Berenberg, M.D., Professor of Pediatrics at Harvard Medical School, whose example instilled in me a love for pediatric neurology and handicapped children;

Dr. T. Barry Brazelton, M.D., Chief of the Division of Child Development and Assoc. Professor of Pediatrics at Harvard Medical School for his encouragement during the preparation of this book;

Dr. Sheldon Simon, M.D., Director of the Gait Laboratory and Assoc. Professor of Orthopedics at Harvard Medical School for showing me that the study of human gait can be fascinating;

Dr. Jon Aagaard, M.D., my dear friend and colleague for constructive criticism and suggestions;

Ms. Joanne Zurek R.N. and Ms. Norma Garvey R.N., for checking the manuscript for accuracy;

Mrs. John Aagaard and Mrs. Jim Milonas for reviewing the book from the parent's viewpoint;

Mr. Paul Mouw for invaluable assistance and advice;

and finally, the parents and their children who in consulting with me over the years, have been my best instructors.

To my wife, my best friend.

Contents

Introduction

Doctor, I took my child to the store for some shoes, and the salesman said he needed orthopedic shoes. But I don't see any problem with his feet. Does he really need orthopedic shoes?

My child has been in-toeing since he started to walk. My pediatrician said he will outgrow it. It's been three years now, and he still in-toes. What should I do?

My three-year-old has mild flatfeet. Last weekend, my husband took him to see a practitioner, who recommended surgery. This was a complete shock to us. So we took him to our pediatrician who suggested we come and talk to you.

Real-life situations like these in my practice prompted me to think seriously about writing a book about children's feet. I wanted something for the parents of young children—many of whom are totally confused by the conflicting advice from pediatricians, family doctors, orthopedic surgeons, podiatrists, chiropractors, grandmothers, aunts, and well-meaning neighbors. What is a parent to do?

I feel that the solution lies in a basic knowledge of children's feet and gait, explained in simple terms, so that a parent with no medical background can understand what is going on with his child's feet. It is not my intention to encourage parents

11

to self-treat their children, but that parents, armed with some understanding of their children's feet and leg problems, may participate more effectively in the health care of their children.

It seems to me that for 50 percent of the patients that I see (and mine is a referral practice; i.e., patients are first seen by a primary care physician) a single session of explaining the child's condition and advice about foot care is all that is needed. An enlightened parent is a satisfied patient. I strongly disagree with those doctors who feel that when parents bring their children in for a consultation, they will not be satisfied until something is prescribed, be it a brace or corrective shoes. I feel that most parents want the best for their children and are intelligent enough to understand that the best, in some instances, may be "masterly neglect."

Occasionally, I have parents who come into my office and demand X rays, braces, or some other kind of treatment they have heard about. Thankfully, such parents are rare. My experience has been that the vast majority of parents come sincerely seeking a truthful answer. A common response after a consultation is, "I'm so relieved. Thanks for taking time to explain this to me."

In this book I will first describe briefly how a normal foot looks and works. Then I will discuss the common foot and leg problems I see in my orthopedic practice, including their diagnosis and treatment. Hopefully, this will give parents some understanding of these conditions, so that when they are confronted with them, they can participate more effectively with the physician in their treatment. Finally, a practical chapter on how to select shoes for children will help parents with this often vexing, yet vital, task.

A word of caution: This book is an expanded version of conversations I have had with parents in the consultation room. It is not an exhaustive treatise on children's feet. You will notice that technical terms have been kept to a minimum; a practical approach has been used throughout, providing the reader with useful information, not theoretical knowledge. This book is not to be used for self-diagnosis and treatment. The contents are solely for educational purposes to encourage more effective parental participation in the doctor's treatment.

During the writing of this book, I initially referred to the parent and the child as "he or she" and "him or her." I was beset with such long and cumbersome sentences that my simple mind was sorely tempted to refer to the child as "it!" However, a flash of ingenuity helped me resolve the problem by referring to the parent as "she" and the child as "he."

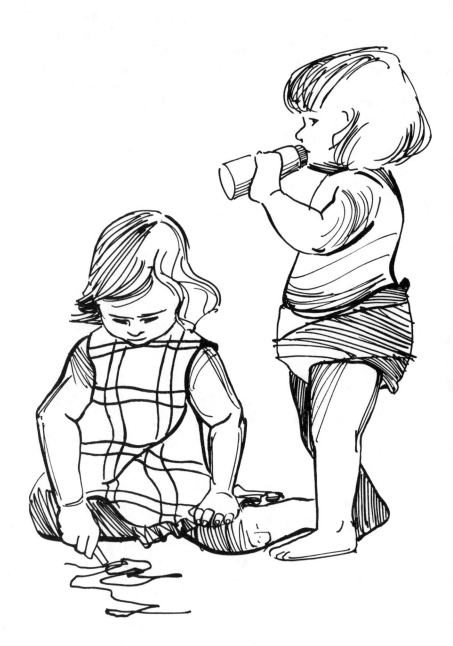

Chapter 1
So, What's Normal?

"Normalcy" is always difficult to define, and so is the normal foot. Does it mean most common? or average? or usual? Does it mean a foot that looks normal? or is pain free on walking? Or does it mean a foot that has no difficulty finding shoes that fit?

Instead of getting mired in theoretical discussions, I will try to describe what a "normal" foot should look like and how it should work.

You may look at your child's feet in many different ways and still not decide if he has normal feet. This may be because you do not know what to look for. Here are several screening tests you can perform on your child that will determine if you should be concerned about his feet.

1. With the child standing, look at his feet from the back. Observe the heel cords (tendo-Achilles) connecting the calves to the heels. They should travel straight up and down, or deviate very slightly outward as they descend from the calves to the heels. Any significant deviation is abnormal.

2. With the child standing, look at the inner (medial) aspects of his feet. Observe the instep, which should be slightly convex upward, representing the longitudinal arch. If the child has a high arch, it is easily observed. But if he has a low arch (which is also normal), it is easily mistaken as flatfeet. The way

15

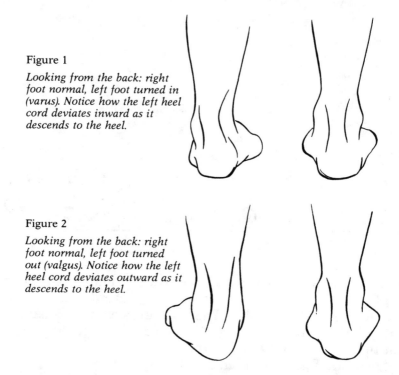

Figure 1

Looking from the back: right foot normal, left foot turned in (varus). Notice how the left heel cord deviates inward as it descends to the heel.

Figure 2

Looking from the back: right foot normal, left foot turned out (valgus). Notice how the left heel cord deviates outward as it descends to the heel.

to identify a low arch is to look for the dark crescentic shadow that indicates that the arch, however low, is present. Up to the age of three years, a low arch is the rule, as chapter 3 will explain.

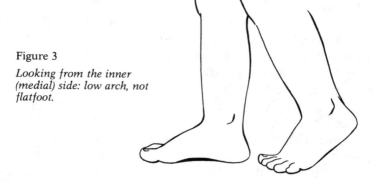

Figure 3

Looking from the inner (medial) side: low arch, not flatfoot.

3. Have the child do a deep knee bend or squat (assuming the child is three or older). This is a very useful test. If he can squat with both feet planted squarely on the ground, his Achilles tendons are adequate and not tight. If the child is able to get up from the squatting to the standing position without help, it indicates good strong quadriceps (thigh) muscles. Since most serious childhood muscle diseases affect the quadriceps before they involve other muscles, strong quadriceps rule out any muscular dystrophy.

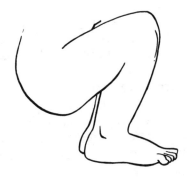

Figure 4

Ability to squat indicates that the Achilles tendons are not tight. Ability to get up from the squatting position without help indicates strong quadriceps muscles and rules out muscular dystrophy.

4. With the child lying down, examine the soles of his feet ("view from the bottom").

Figure 5

View from the bottom. The imaginary axis (central line) should fall between the second and third toes in a normal foot. Any deviation indicates forefoot deformity.

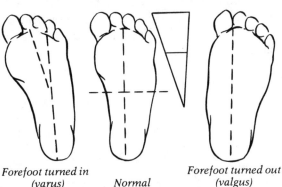

Forefoot turned in (varus)   *Normal*   *Forefoot turned out (valgus)*

The foot consists of the hindfoot and the forefoot. Imagine the hindfoot as being in the shape of a triangle and the forefoot a trapezoid. The trapezoid should be connected to the triangle squarely, with no marked deviation in either direction. If you draw an imaginary axis (central line) from the tip of the heel posteriorly to the toes anteriorly, it should roughly bisect the foot into two approximately equal halves. You have to realize, of course, that we are talking in approximate terms, since the foot is not exactly symmetrical.

Check the inner and outer borders of the foot. They meet at the heel posteriorly, and run straight forward, but deviating from each other. The outer border should be perfectly straight, although the inner border is slightly curved due to the longitudinal arch.

If the forefoot deviates inward in relation to the hindfoot, the foot is said to be in *varus* or *adductus*. If the forefoot is deviated outward in relation to the hindfoot, the foot is in *valgus*. But more of this in chapter 2.

5. Look at the child walk, first away from you and then toward you. Observe the direction of his feet: Do they turn in or out? The normal gait should be smoothly executed, with no jerky movements, and the feet should be pointed straight ahead or slightly outward. If the feet turn in or out excessively, refer to chapter 2 for an explanation.

Observe the child as he takes a step forward. Does the forward foot hit the ground with the heel, or with the toes? In the normal heel-toe gait, the heel is the first part of the foot to hit the ground, followed by the rest of the foot and the toes. If the toes hit the ground before the heel, the child may have tight heel cords. A full discussion of this subject is provided in chapter 3.

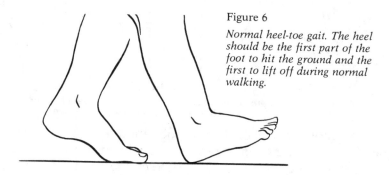

Figure 6

Normal heel-toe gait. The heel should be the first part of the foot to hit the ground and the first to lift off during normal walking.

This, then, is a screening procedure any parent can use on her child. As later chapters will indicate, children go through different phases of skeletal growth; many "deformities" observed in childhood are often just normal variations that correct spontaneously with time. The parent who has taken the time to educate herself in these matters will save herself a lot of unnecessary concern when she sees her child with these "deformities." On the other hand, if the child does have a problem that requires medical intervention, she will be able to participate more effectively with the physician in the care of the child.

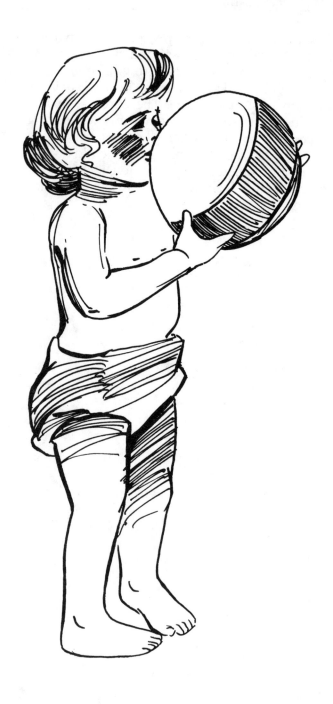

Chapter 2
Toe In, Toe Out

Toe In

Because toeing in (or pigeon-toed) is by far commoner than toeing out, we will discuss it first.

Not infrequently, confused and bewildered mothers come into my office because of the conflicting opinions that had been offered by various people from grandmothers to pediatricians regarding their children's in-toeing. Some mothers are frustrated to the verge of tears.

The reason for this confusion is that in-toeing is often taken (even among professionals) to be a diagnosis rather than a symptom. Let me explain what I mean by this.

Your child has a fever, so you take him to the doctor. He sticks a thermometer in the child's mouth, very wisely confirms that he does have a fever, prescribes some aspirin and leaves the room. Would you be happy with the visit? Of course not! You would ask, "But Doctor, what is causing the fever? Don't you want to check his throat, his ears, his lungs to see what is causing the fever?"

In the same way, when you bring your child to the doctor because he is pigeon-toed, and the doctor watches him walk, agrees that he is indeed pigeon-toed, and prescribes his favorite treatment for in-toeing (be it shoes or braces or nothing), he has not even begun to address the problem. The question the doctor has to ask himself is, What is causing the in-toeing? Until the answer is found, the proper treatment for that child cannot be prescribed.

There are three primary causes of in-toeing in a child. The problem could be in the feet, the legs, or the hips. The treatment of in-toeing should therefore be directed toward the cause of the in-toeing, not the symptom of in-toeing.

The three primary causes of in-toeing are: (1) metatarsus adductus (in the feet); (2) internal tibial torsion (in the legs); (3) femoral torsion (at the hips).

Metatarsus Adductus

If you look at the bottom of the foot of a newborn, you will notice a gradual curvature in the inner border of the foot. This

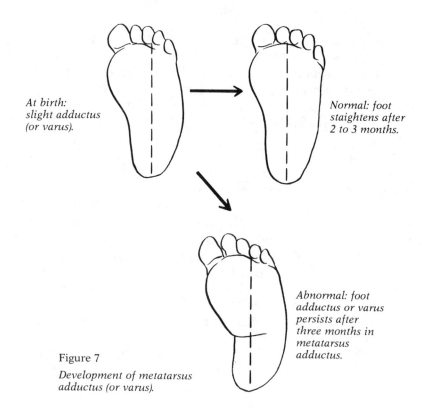

At birth: slight adductus (or varus).

Normal: foot staightens after 2 to 3 months.

Abnormal: foot adductus or varus persists after three months in metatarsus adductus.

Figure 7

Development of metatarsus adductus (or varus).

is normal and is not to be confused with any foot deformity. By the time the baby reaches three months of age, the foot should straighten out on its own. If, after three months, the foot still turns in significantly, corrective measures are needed.

Metatarsus adductus (MTA) or metatarsus varus is a condition in which the forefoot is turned in (adducted) in relation to the hindfoot. This is easily seen by looking at the bottom of the foot. Very often, there is a crease at the midpoint of the inner border of the foot, between the forefoot and hindfoot where the turning in occurs.

The cause of the condition is persistence of the turned-in position of the feet as they were held in the womb, although genetic factors may also be involved. It is an extremely common condition, being present in 70 percent of all babies at birth. Fortunately, most of these straighten out in the first six to twelve weeks of life.

The usual treatment for this condition is manipulation and casting in the office by a trained, experienced physician. Six weeks of casting is usually required. Because the casts fit tightly, they have to be changed at two-week intervals. Once correction has been obtained, the feet can be held in the corrected position with outflare shoes for two to three months. On this treatment regime, results are usually excellent with very little recurrence.

Shoes alone may be adequate for a very mild case of MTA, but in most cases serial casting is necessary. This is because shoes do not correct the deformity; they only hold the correction, once it has been obtained.

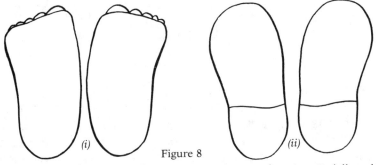

Figure 8

Treatment of metatarsus adductus consists of repeated castings (i), followed by wearing of outflare shoes (ii).

What if the deformity is left alone even after three months? No one knows for sure. Several long-term studies and most orthopedists agree that some children will improve spontaneously. However, in many of these children, a significant deformity persists, giving rise to cosmetic and functional problems like bunions and difficulty fitting shoes.

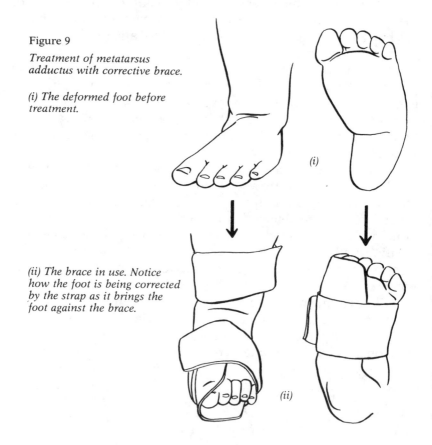

Figure 9

Treatment of metatarsus adductus with corrective brace.

(i) The deformed foot before treatment.

(ii) The brace in use. Notice how the foot is being corrected by the strap as it brings the foot against the brace.

More recently, in an attempt to avoid the inconvenience and emotional grief inflicted on both parent and child by repeated castings, I have developed a corrective brace for metatarsus adductus which can be used as an alternative to casting. The most attractive feature of the brace is convenience. It may be removed twice a day for cleaning, and any skin problems are avoided. The average duration of bracing to obtain correction has been about three months. The brace has been extensively tested in the last three years, and now accepted as an effective alternative to repeated castings in metatarsus adductus. Named the Wheaton brace™, it is now being used by orthopedic surgeons across North America and Europe.

Congenital Clubfoot

Congenital clubfoot (or more properly called congenital talipes equino-varus) is not one of the common causes of in-toeing. But I would like to discuss it after MTA, because, like MTA, there is adduction of the foot. However, it is a much more serious condition than MTA.

In MTA the forefoot is turned in but the hindfoot is in a perfectly normal position. In clubfoot both the forefoot and the hindfoot are turned in severely. Moreover, the heel cord is markedly shortened so that the foot points downward (the equinus deformity) as well as inward (the varus deformity). Hence the child has a severe deformity where the foot is pointed downward and twisted inward so that the sole of the foot is facing inward rather than downward (the equino-varus deformity). These deformities are fixed or rigid; the foot cannot be pushed or twisted back into the normal position.

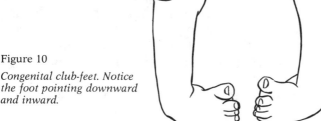

Figure 10

Congenital club-feet. Notice the foot pointing downward and inward.

The cause of this condition is not entirely understood, although genetic factors are definitely involved. Disturbance of foot development very early in pregnancy somehow causes the tendons and ligaments on the inner side of the foot to underdevelop. These underdeveloped ligaments and tendons tend to be tight (contractured) and pull the foot into the characteristic equino-varus deformity just described. By the time of birth, the deformity is already well established.

Treatment of this condition has to be vigorous and prompt. The recommended treatment is manipulation and repeated casting of the foot as soon as possible after birth. Doctors jest about the breech baby with clubfeet doing better than the baby that presents headfirst because the doctor could start casting the clubfeet while waiting for the head. This just underscores the need for prompt treatment.

Treatment for clubfoot is a prolonged process. Repeated casting—weekly at first and every other week after that—is required for a period of three to six months. In those children fortunate enough to respond to casting alone, corrective shoes (called tarso-pronator shoes) are worn full-time for at least one year. This is because recurrence is such a common problem in the first year of life, even after a favorable response to casting.

In about half the children with clubfeet, casting alone is not sufficient to correct the deformities completely. One or more surgical procedures are required to lengthen or release the tight tendons and ligaments. Following these surgical procedures, more casting is usually required.

It cannot be over stressed that, unlike MTA, clubfoot is a potentially crippling condition which, if left untreated, could cause misery to the child. Fortunately, it is rare and does not constitute a major cause of in-toeing. If you have a child with clubfoot, do not feel overwhelmed. It can be helped, and surgical correction often restores the feet to near normal. But you would need to thoroughly discuss your child's problem with your doctor. Don't hesitate to ask him all the questions you have. He must explain things to you, even if the results of his treatment might not be as ideal as you both may want it to be.

Internal Tibial Torsion

When you look at the soles of your child's feet ("view from the bottom"), you may be satisfied that the infant does not have metatarsus adductus or clubfoot. But you may be disturbed to find that he is nevertheless pigeon-toed. Why is this?

If your child is less than eighteen months of age, the problem is probably due to a common condition called internal tibial torsion (ITT). This condition is so common that it is considered normal in the first year of the child's life (if by "normal" is meant "the majority").

The way to check for ITT is to have the child lie on his back and flex his knees, keeping his kneecaps (patellae) facing you squarely. If the child has ITT, you will find the foot (or feet, depending on whether it's affecting one or both legs) pointing inward toward the midline rather than straight forward. The problem is not in the feet (you have previously ascertained that), but in the leg bones (tibia and fibula). The leg bones are twisted inward (intorsion) so that the transverse axes of the knees and ankle are at right angles to each other.

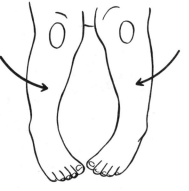

Figure 11

Internal tibial torsion. Notice that the patellae (kneecaps) are facing forward, indicating that the twisting occurs in the leg bones below the level of the knees.

This deformity is due to the position of the legs in the womb. As the child develops, the twisting (or intorsion) tends to correct itself. By the time the child reaches his first birthday and starts to walk, the bones have untwisted themselves, and the child walks with his feet pointing straight ahead or slightly outward. However, if the deformity persists, then the act of walking will make it obvious for the first time, since he now walks pigeon-toed. If such a child also happened to have MTA and was treated by casting and declared "cured," this could be very distressing to the parents, who fear a recurrence of MTA. This could be easily avoided if the doctor who had treated the child for MTA had warned the parents about ITT.

ITT does not require any treatment for the first twelve to fifteen months of life; 95 percent of the cases resolve spontaneously. However, if after this age the deformity persists and is severe, corrective measures may be indicated. The traditional method of treatment for ITT has been the use of the Fillauer bar (or splint), which clamps onto the shoes in the externally rotated (rolled-out) position. A similar bar called the Denis-Browne splint is screwed onto the shoes rather than clamped on, but the principle is the same. This is applied at bedtime and it is worn for an average of nine to twelve months.

I have not been happy with the shoes and bar method of treatment. With both feet clamped together it is very confining and not well tolerated. It seems like severe punishment

Figure 12

Fillauer bar in use, typically at bedtime between one and two years of age, with the legs rotated outward 35 degrees.

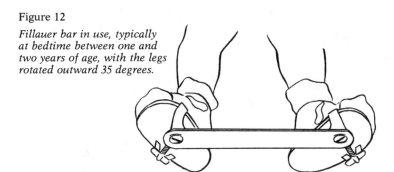

for a fairly innocuous condition. Moreover, the use of shoes and bar for tibial torsion is conceptually unsound. Since the knees are held extended during treatment, any rotation force applied is transmitted to the hip rather than on the tibia where the corrective torque is desired.

For these reasons the shoes and bar method of treatment has fallen out of favor with many physicians. In recent years, I have been using a device called the Telescoping Brace that

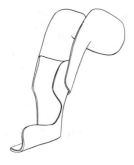

Figure 12A
*The Telescoping Brace for
the right leg.*

holds the knee in flexion, thereby directing the corrective torque on the tibia where it is needed. Moreover, it is much less confining and hence well tolerated by patients. It comes ready-made in several sizes, and used for night wear only. Average time in brace required for correction has been about three months, although I keep the child on the brace at night for a total of six months to prevent recurrence.

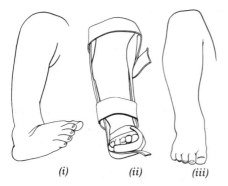

Figure 12B
*Treatment of Internal
Tibial Torsion
(i)Before Treatment
(ii)In Telescoping Brace
(iii)After night bracing for
3 months*

(i)   (ii)   (iii)

What is the optimal time for the treatment of tibial torsion? Some physicians prescribe treatment from the age of three months. Understanding the natural history of this condition will lead one to reject this approach. On the other hand, some physicians believe ITT should never be treated. Their approach stems from the conviction that ITT always corrects spontaneously and that no conclusive study gives a clear indication of the best treatment. The truth of the matter is that no one knows for sure.

In my practice I have time and again consulted with parents who brought their children to my office because of persistent in-toeing from ITT. They had been assured by their physicians that there was nothing to worry about. They watched their children in-toe year after year. Some of these children were four or five years of age. What could one say to such parents?

Recognizing that most ITT's will improve spontaneously by the age of twelve to fifteen months, I would certainly not treat ITT before this age. If the ITT remains significant by the time children are toddlers, I start them on the Telescoping Brace at night. When I was using the shoes and bar, there was a sense of urgency with treatment, because beyond the age of two years patient acceptance was virtually nil. Hence it was important to get treatment started by eighteen months of age. With the Telescoping Brace that I now use, there is no longer that sense of urgency. In borderline cases, I can safely observe them beyond two years of age. I have effectively used the Telescoping Brace on children two to three years of age with excellent patient acceptance.

Femoral Torsion

You may have a child who does not appear to have MTA or ITT, but who still in-toes. It is likely that he is a child between the ages of three and eight. You may notice that he in-toes when he walks or trips frequently due to the in-toeing. He might even have had treatment for MTA and ITT in the past, and you begin to wonder what has gone wrong.

The most probable cause of in-toeing in such a situation is not a recurrence of previous problems, but a condition called femoral torsion. Just as the tibia could be twisted inward producing tibial torsion, the femur could also be twisted inward. Most of the twisting occurs at the upper end of the femur at the hip.

This condition is present at birth, but it is usually not evident until the age of three or four years. By then, the tibial torsion (ITT) has resolved, and the effect of the femoral torsion is unmasked.

You will notice that, as the child walks toward you, his kneecaps squint inward with each step. This indicates that the twisting is occurring above the knees at the hips rather than below the knees (as in ITT).

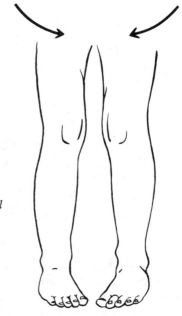

Figure 13

Femoral torsion. Notice the patellae (kneecaps) squinting inward, indicating that the twisting occurs above the level of the knees, near the hips.

When he is reminded, the child could deliberately rotate his legs out and walk reasonably straight. However, toward the evening when his muscles are tired and unable to compensate, his feet will turn in. If for some reason he is wearing heavy orthopedic shoes, the shoes will act as pendulums, pulling his feet into the in-toeing position.

Doctors (especially orthopedists) may call femoral torsion by another name: excessive femoral anteversion. This term more accurately describes the phenomenon, but it is less easily understood.

Let's look at the anatomy of the hip joint. It consists of a ball (the femoral head) and a socket (the acetabular cup). The ball points inward and 15 degrees forward, articulating with the socket in a snug fit.

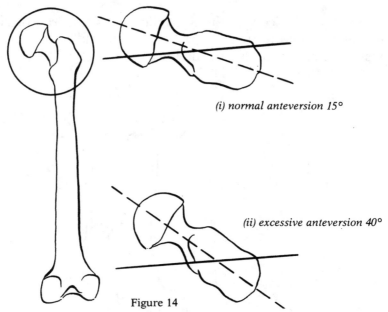

(i) normal anteversion 15°

(ii) excessive anteversion 40°

Figure 14

Femoral anteversion. Notice the femoral head pointing inward and forward at an angle of 15° in (i) and 40° in (ii).

This slightly forward projection of the femoral head and neck is the normal femoral anteversion seen in older children and adults. At birth, femoral anteversion is measured at 40 degrees. This angle rapidly decreases as the child grows. By the age of eight, the normal adult anteversion angle of 15 degrees is obtained. In most children, this is a smooth and consistent decrease, with no postural or gait problem. In some children, however, the anteversion angle of 40 degrees present at birth persists into early and even later childhood. To keep the femoral head in the socket, the whole lower limb rotates or twists inward, giving the appearance of in-toeing when the child walks.

The way to demonstrate excessive femoral anteversion on your child is to have him lie on his stomach. With both knees flexed at 90 degrees, and both legs pointing straight toward the ceiling, externally and internally rotate the hips, using the legs as the levers going through the arc of rotation. In a child with normal femoral anteversion, both external and internal rotation should be almost equal; in a child with excessive femoral anteversion, the range of internal rotation far exceeds that of external rotation.

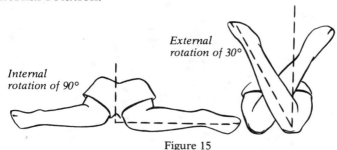

Figure 15

Test to demonstrate excessive femoral anteversion (femoral torsion). Internal rotation is far in excess of external rotation.

It used to be fashionable for doctors to put these children in corrective shoes with wedges, braces, and twister cables. Recent verifiable studies have demonstrated that none of these cumbersome treatment regimes influence to any significant degree the outcome of the problem.

Femoral torsion corrects itself with time. Practically all children with this problem walk straight by their eighth birthday.

Understanding the natural history of this condition helps you to participate in any management decisions regarding your child. My advice to any parent who brings her child in for this condition is as follows:

1. Encourage the child to sit cross-legged (Indian style or tailor's position) as soon as he is old enough to do so. I would actively discourage the child from sitting on his knees or his feet, in the so-called W-position (or reversed tailor's position). Sitting on his feet or knees tends to perpetuate the problem of excessive femoral anteversion, whereas sitting cross-legged reverses the deformity and encourages resolution of the problem.

Why do some children sit in the W-position but have no in-toeing problem? This posture does not *cause* in-toeing, it only *perpetuates* it. If a child is structurally normal to begin with, sitting on his knees or feet does no harm. However, if the child

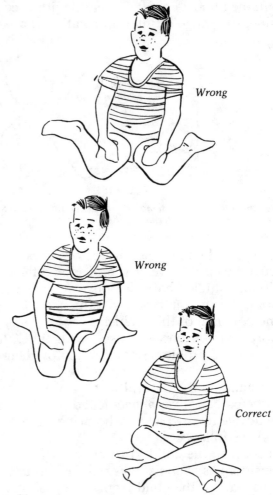

Figure 16
Proper and improper sitting positions

has excessive femoral anteversion, he will tend to sit on his knees or his feet due to the turned-in position of his legs. In so doing, he perpetuates the deformity.

2. Assure the parents that this condition will resolve, but that it takes time: YEARS. By the time the child reaches his eighth birthday, the problem will have resolved. It is very im-

portant for parents to understand this, otherwise they will fall prey to unsound advice (professional or otherwise) and end up with all kinds of expensive shoes and braces.

What if the problem is not resolved even after the child is eight years old? To assure parents, I have only to cite the large number of children, followed up over many years, who corrected themselves completely. In those few where the correction is not complete, the residual deformity is so mild that it is hardly noticeable. The exceptions are children with cerebral palsy or other forms of severe paralysis. The femoral torsion in these children tends to persist, and bracing or even surgery may be required. For otherwise normal children, I repeat that braces and corrective shoes are unnecessary and possibly harmful.

In summary, in-toeing is a symptom and can be due to one of three major causes: metatarsus adductus, internal tibial torsion, or femoral torsion. Each of these conditions should be approached differently. Both the physician and parent should be clear in their minds what is causing the in-toeing and direct their treatment to the cause, not the symptom, of in-toeing.

Toe Out

Toeing out, though less commonly seen in the office, is nevertheless a frequently encountered problem. This condition is most common among young infants. The three primary causes of toeing out are: (1) postural calcaneo-valgus (in the feet); (2) external tibial torsion (in the legs); (3) external rotatory contracture (at the hips).

Postural Calcaneo-Valgus

This common problem is evident at birth and can appear very alarming. The deformity is opposite to that of a clubfoot; the whole foot is turned up and outward, touching the lower part of the shin.

However, unlike clubfoot, the deformity is not rigid. Gentle but firm pressure corrects the deformity and allows the foot to assume a more normal position, if only momentarily. If the

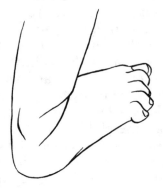

Figure 17

Calcaneo-valgus in an infant. The whole foot is turned upward and outward, touching the lower part of the shin.

child is otherwise normal with no other problems, one can confidently expect this condition to completely correct itself in six to nine months. Gentle manipulation by the parent at home with each diaper change may hasten the time taken for resolution of the problem. Casting is rarely necessary, and only in the extreme case.

A much rarer but more serious and rigid variety of calcaneo-valgus may occur in isolation, but it is usually associated with serious paralytic conditions like spina bifida. Aggressive casting and surgery may be needed in those cases.

External Tibial Torsion

This is the opposite deformity to the much more common internal tibial torsion (ITT) that we discussed earlier. Like ITT, it tends to improve spontaneously by the age of one year. If the problem is severe after the age of one, use of a Telescoping brace may be required with the legs held in the neutral position. I have never had to treat such a case, and the experience with this problem by other orthopedic surgeons is very limited.

External Rotatory Contracture

In this case the infant appears at birth with external rotation of the entire lower limb, so that the foot is pointing outward almost perpendicular to the body. This condition is thought to be due to tightness of the posterior structures of the hip (the buttock muscles). This condition usually corrects itself as the child begins to walk, and after the age of one, the problem gradually disappears. Stretching exercises by rolling both legs inward may help, though the efficacy of such exercises has not been proven.

Generally, toeing out due to whatever condition in an otherwise healthy child does not need therapeutic intervention, since it corrects itself after the age of one. Toeing in, on the other hand, is much more common and may require corrective treatment in some cases.

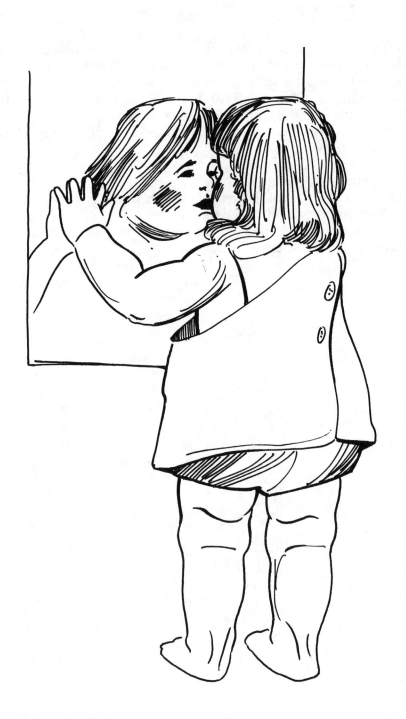

Chapter 3
A Matter of Arches

The upright posture in humans demands that the foot provide a stable, adaptable base for support and a flexible lever for propulsion in ambulation. For both these functions, the foot is constructed perfectly. A series of bones held together by resilient ligaments and powered by strong muscles and tendons, the foot is truly a remarkable piece of engineering.

A distinct example of how the foot's structure is uniquely suited to its function is shown by the longitudinal arch of the foot. Architecturally speaking, the arch enables the foot to give more support per given amount of structural material than any

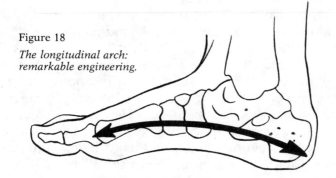

Figure 18

The longitudinal arch: remarkable engineering.

other type of construction. In fact, the unique arrangement of the bones with the ligaments forming the arch is so stable that the muscles of the foot do no work in the standing position. That is why one can stand for long periods of time with ease.

Everyone agrees that the arch is important. But the consensus among professionals breaks down when it comes to dealing with a child with no foot arch, i.e., flatfeet.

A recent survey of orthopedic surgeons, pediatric orthopedists, pediatricians, and podiatrists (all people who dole out advice about feet problems) indicated wide differences of opinion regarding both the need for treatment as well as the modes of treatment. These differences of opinions were not just between the different groups (e.g., orthopedic surgeons vs. podiatrists), but within each group as well. Treatment preferences ranged from no treatment for flatfeet, to use of corrective shoes and arch supports, to surgical correction. No wonder the parent is confused!

A great deal of the confusion lies in the fact that people are not defining flatfeet specifically enough to allow for any meaningful comparison of results of treatment modalities. The basic thing to realize about flatfeet is that there are different kinds of flatfeet: *apparent or actual, flexible or rigid.*

By flatfeet most people mean the absence of a normal arch in the child's feet while he is standing. In a child under the age of two years, this is almost always the case. The arch is obscured at this age by the presence of a pad of fat in that area of the foot, making the foot appear flat. However, if you move the joints of the foot, the foot is perfectly flexible in all directions. Therefore, before the age of three years, if the child is otherwise healthy and the feet are flexible and painless, absolutely nothing should be done for the "flatfeet."

The arch becomes more obvious when the child reaches the age of three, as the fat pad of infancy disappears. If you examine the feet of a child while he is sitting or lying down, you will usually see a well-formed arch. However, as soon as he stands up, the arches seem to disappear under the weight of his body. Parents sometimes consider this as being "flat-footed," and they get unduly concerned. However, if they look closely enough, they may see a small crescentic shadow under the instep, indicating that the child has low arches. Low arches are perfectly normal, and do not require any treatment.

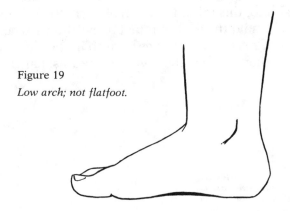

Figure 19
Low arch; not flatfoot.

Some children, however, are truly flat-footed. If you look at the inner border of the foot on standing, it appears flat or even slightly bulging where the arch should be. Looking at his heels from the back, the tendo-Achilles deviates outward excessively as it descends to the heel.

Figure 20

True flexible flatfeet:
(i) Looking from the inner (medial) side, the lower border of the foot is completely flat. (ii) Looking from the back, the tendo-Achilles deviates outward as it descends to the heel.

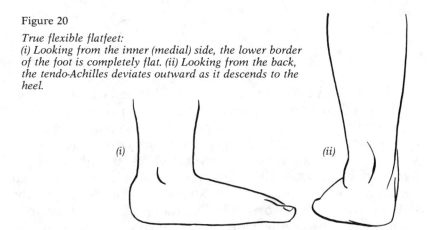

(i)   *(ii)*

This is *true flexible flatfeet*. They are flexible in that as soon as the foot is not bearing weight, the arch reappears. True flexible or postural flatfeet, though usually not a serious condition, runs in families. The condition does require support. In a growing child, this takes the form of corrective shoes with arch supports to hold the arches intact as he stands. The shoes hold the bones of his feet that form the arch in the right relationship to one another, so that they will not be misshapen.

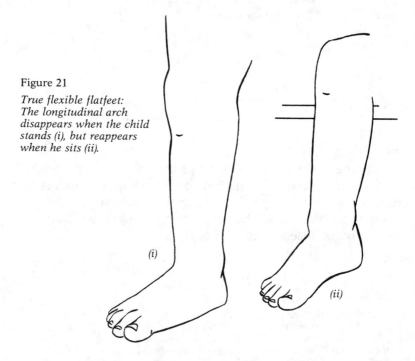

Figure 21

True flexible flatfeet: The longitudinal arch disappears when the child stands (i), but reappears when he sits (ii).

(i)

(ii)

I ordinarily prescribe oxfords (laced shoes) with inner heel wedges and soft arch supports. Others may prefer more rigid arch supports. In any case, the parent should understand that arch supports and corrective shoes do not *cure* flatfeet. After wearing corrective shoes for several years (usually until the age of eight), most of these children are still flat-footed. What the arch supports and corrective shoes have done is prevent the flatfeet from getting worse. Flexible flatfeet, in most instances, do not cause problems. Only the extreme cases develop foot strain or pain during prolonged walking. Hopefully, the corrective shoes and arch supports will prevent this from happening.

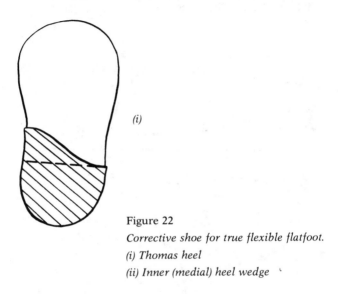

(i)

Figure 22
Corrective shoe for true flexible flatfoot.
(i) Thomas heel
(ii) Inner (medial) heel wedge

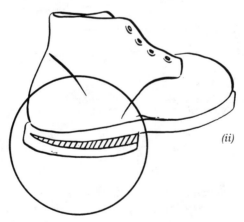

(ii)

A small group of flexible (or postural) flatfeet also have associated tight tendo-Achilles. This can be determined by attempting to flex the foot upward at the ankle, while keeping the knee straight. Normally, the foot could dorsiflex to 20 degrees beyond neutral. In a child with tight heel cords, the foot could not be dorsiflexed to the neutral position.

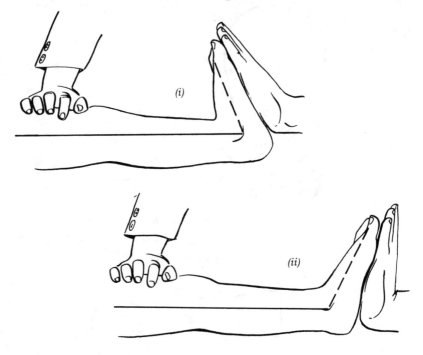

Figure 23

Testing for tendo-Achilles tightness.
(i) Normal—the foot could dorsiflex to 20°
beyond neutral.
(ii) Tight tendo-Achilles—the foot could not be
dorsiflexed to the neutral position.

Heel cord stretching exercises at home, or even physical therapy, may be required in these children to overcome the tightness. A plastic brace (ankle-foot orthosis) may also be helpful in keeping the foot in the neutral position.

In young children, there is a rare form of flatfoot which is rigid. This appears at birth and is often associated with severe neurological or muscular disease. The foot is completely flat, in fact, convex downward even without weightbearing. This gives a rounded appearance to the bottom of the foot, hence the name "rocker-bottom foot." The cause is dislocation of the talus in utero, and the condition is called *congenital vertical talus*. This condition requires aggressive casting and surgical correction early in life. Fortunately, it is an extremely rare disease.

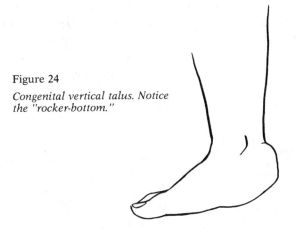

Figure 24

Congenital vertical talus. Notice the "rocker-bottom."

Flatfeet accompanied by pain occurs only in older children after the age of six. This is usually due to muscle spasm from injury or an underlying bone or joint problem, as in *Kohler's disease* (inflammation of the navicular bone in the foot), tarsal coalition (where two or more bones of the foot are fused together abnormally at birth, but do not get painful until the child is about ten years old), or an *accessory navicular bone* (an extra piece of loose bone at the instep where a tendon inserts). Without going into the details of these conditions, suffice it to say that flatfeet associated with pain should always be seen by a doctor.

The Role of Surgery in Flatfeet

In cases of congenital vertical talus and some cases of painful flatfeet mentioned above, surgery is necessary. But what about the common, painless, flexible flatfeet that we discussed earlier? Is there a place for surgery?

On several occasions parents have come to my office for a consultation because surgery has been recommended for their child's flatfeet by someone else. I always explain to them that the attitude toward surgery for flexible (postural) flatfeet has evolved significantly in recent years from one of enthusiasm to skepticism—and for good reason. Most of the surgical procedures devised in the past have not withstood the test of time; many of them are not based on sound biomechanical principles, and are essentially obsolete. (An example of such a procedure is arthroeresis, in which the stem of a silastic implant is inserted on the subtalar joint to prevent progression of flexible flatfeet. And to think that such a procedure was advocated as prophylaxis in children as young as two is horrifying!)

Two surgical procedures are reasonable to do when indicated: (1) heel cord lengthening when the heel cords are tight, and (2) calaneal osteotomy (cutting the calcaneus bone) to realign the subtalar joint. Fusions of the bones of the feet, which were in vogue in the 60's and early 70's, are now rarely done. Long-term follow-up studies have shown rapidly deteriorating results over time.

While it may still be necessary for an adult with severe flatfeet to have surgery because of pain, young children with flexible flatfeet are not candidates for surgery. If surgery is even mentioned for your child in such a context, please get a second opinion.

The Role of Exercise in Flatfeet

Some practitioners prescribe foot exercises for flatfeet. They feel that stronger muscles would somehow support the foot bones better and restore the longitudinal arches to the feet. However, recent studies have shown that the stability of the arch depends on the shape of the bones and the support of the ligaments. Laxity of the ligaments allows for loss of the arch at a young age. If left unsupported, the bones develop in this abnormal position, become misshapen and perpetuate the flat-footedness. Hence it is important in true flexible flatfeet to support the arches with corrective shoes and arch supports.

The muscles of the foot play no part in maintaining the arch during normal standing. Electromyographic studies recently demonstrated that there is no electrical activity in the muscles of the foot when one is standing still. Therefore, exercises, try as you may, will not restore your child's arches if he does not already possess them.

In summary, some flatfeet in young children are of the flexible or postural kind. Some are not true flatfeet, but merely low arches where no treatment is required. In those with true flexible flatfeet, corrective shoes and arch supports may be helpful in preventing progression, but they are not curative. Surgery is unnecessary, and foot exercises are not helpful. On the other hand, flatfeet which are rigid or painful are more serious and need medical evaluation and treatment.

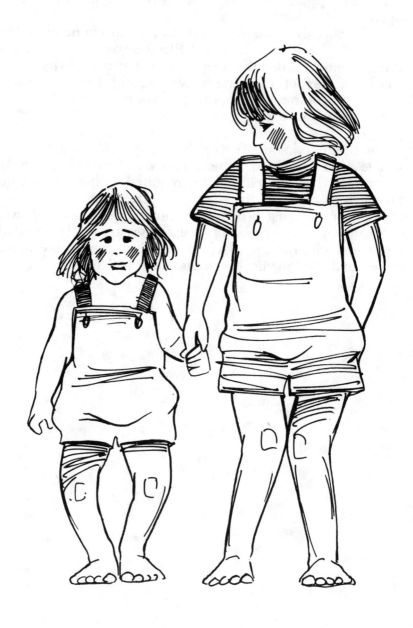

Chapter 4
Bowlegs and Knock-knees

In chapter 2 we discussed toe in and toe out which are rotational problems of the lower limbs. In this chapter we will discuss angular problems: bowlegs and knock-knees.

It is important to understand that growth of the bones in the lower limbs occurs at both ends of each bone; i.e., around the hips, the knees, and the ankles. However, 70 percent of the growth occurs around the knees at the lower end of the femur (thigh bone) and the upper end of the tibia (leg bone). As the potential for growth is great, so is the potential for deformity. Any disturbance of growth around the knee gives rise to significant deformities.

If you think of the growth plate (epiphyseal plate) as the site of bone formation, a disturbance to any portion of the epiphyseal plate results in failure of bone growth in that area. If the medial (inner) part of the epiphyseal plate is affected, bone growth is slowed down or stopped in that area. This causes the lateral (outer) parts of the femur and tibia to become longer than the medial parts. These bones therefore curve inward as they grow, resulting in varus or bowing. If bone growth in the lateral portion of the epiphyseal plate of the femur or tibia is slowed down or stopped, then the bones grow in a curved direction outward, resulting in valgus (knock-knees).

49

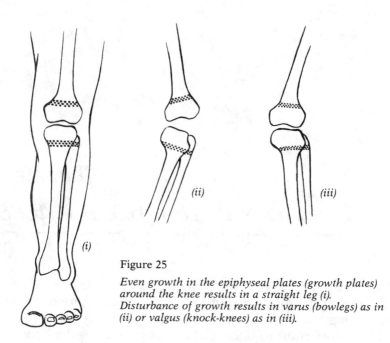

Figure 25

Even growth in the epiphyseal plates (growth plates) around the knee results in a straight leg (i).
Disturbance of growth results in varus (bowlegs) as in (ii) or valgus (knock-knees) as in (iii).

Due to the differential growth of the medial and lateral parts of the epiphyseal plates around the knee in the first few years of life, the normal infant is bowlegged (more properly called *genu varum*) as he starts life in the upright position. This continues until the age of two, when the knees straighten up. However, by the age of three, he starts to develop the opposite "deformity": knock-knees (or *genu valgum*). Left alone, this also corrects spontaneously by the time the child reaches his fifth birthday.

These conditions are usually so mild that most parents do not even notice them. However, some children can get quite bowlegged or knock-kneed and still be within normal limits. Depending on the appearance of the deformity and the sensitivity of the parents, the "problem" can get quite alarming. These conditions can be exaggerated by any rotational problems the child may have at that time (in-toeing or out-toeing). Internal tibial torsion exaggerates any bowleggedness that may be present, while out-toeing exaggerates any knock-knee de-

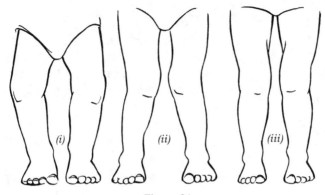

Figure 26

Bowlegs (i) and knock-knees (ii) could be just part of the normal evolution that takes place with growth. The final product at age 5 (iii).

formity. The question facing parents is, When is the condition a problem, or when should a doctor be consulted?

The first thing parents need to learn is how to assess the severity of the bowleggedness or knock-knee deformity.

To measure the amount of bowing, one should first eliminate the rotational component by having the child lie flat on his back with both legs extended and feet pointing directly upward toward the ceiling. Bring the ankles together, and measure the space between the inner borders of both knees. This is known as the intercondylar distance (IC distance).

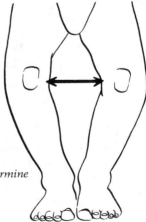

Figure 27

Measuring the intercondylar distance to determine the severity of bowlegs.

To measure the severity of knock-knee deformity, one should first eliminate the rotational component by having the child lie flat with both legs extended, and both kneecaps pointing upward toward the ceiling. The space between the inner ankle bones (medial malleoli) is the intermalleolar distance (IM distance) and gives an objective measurement of the severity of the problem.

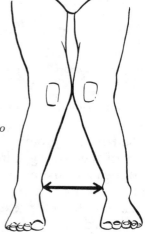

Figure 28

Measuring the intermalleolar distance to determine the severity of knock-knees.

Parents who are concerned about their children in this respect could measure and hence gauge the severity of the deformity and follow its progression, if any, every three months. The intercondylar distance for bowlegs and the intermalleolar distance for knock-knees should not in any case exceed two inches up to the age of five years. A medical consultation should be sought under the following circumstances:

1. The IC distance or IM distance exceeds two inches.

2. Rapid progression of the IC or IM measurement over a six-month period; i.e., more than one-half inch progression.

3. Persistent and obvious deformity beyond the age of two years for bowlegs and beyond the age of five years for knock-knees.

I feel that parents can competently assess their children's

problem this way because practically all these deformities correct spontaneously. In most cases, bracing and corrective shoes are unnecessary and possibly harmful.

What happens when the child's condition goes beyond the prescribed limits mentioned above? He should be evaluated by a doctor. This does not mean that he will need any active treatment. In most cases, observation is all that is needed. However, it is wise under those circumstances to have a professional observe the child with you, in case he develops one of the following rather rare problems.

Severe genu valgus (physiologic). Knock-knees in children up to the age of five years could be safely ignored. If it continues after the age of seven and remains severe, an X ray of the knees should be taken. An X ray picture gives a more accurate evaluation of the severity of knock-knee deformity by measuring the tibio-femoral angle. Under normal circumstances, after the age of seven years, the tibio-femoral angle should not exceed 10 degrees of valgus. (7 degrees is the mean.)

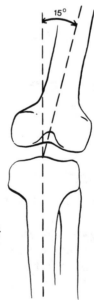

Figure 29

Severe knock-knee deformity. The tibio-femoral angle on X ray picture measures 15°.

If the tibio-femoral angle as measured on X rays is more than 15 degrees valgus and continues to be severe, problems with awkward gait and patellar subluxation may arise in the future. Treatment may therefore be required to correct the deformity. Unfortunately, braces do not help. Surgery becomes necessary by the age of eleven or twelve years.

The most effective way to correct the knock-knee deformity is called epiphyseal stapling. Several large staples are inserted across the epiphyseal plates on the medial (inner) sides, at the lower ends of the tibia and femur. The rationale of the operation is to slow down the growth of the medial portion of the growth plates, thereby allowing the lateral portions to catch up. The staples are removed after a few years once the deformity has been corrected. Results of this operation are good.

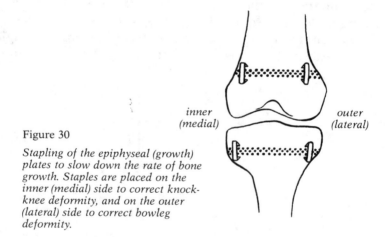

inner
(medial)

outer
(lateral)

Figure 30

Stapling of the epiphyseal (growth) plates to slow down the rate of bone growth. Staples are placed on the inner (medial) side to correct knock-knee deformity, and on the outer (lateral) side to correct bowleg deformity.

Blount's disease. This is a disease that usually affects young black children. The medial part of the growth plate of the tibia fails to develop. The cause of this is not known, but the result is that the knees develop a varus (bowleg) deformity. In the first three years of life this is difficult to diagnose, even with X rays, although the severity of the bowing from infancy raises one's suspicion. Braces have been tried, but their efficacy is dubious.

By the age of three years, if the tibio-femoral angle measures more than 15 degrees, the most effective treatment is surgery. The operation is called corrective osteotomy, correcting the deformity in the upper tibia. Recurrence of the deformity even after osteotomy is not uncommon, and repeated osteotomies are necessary in some children.

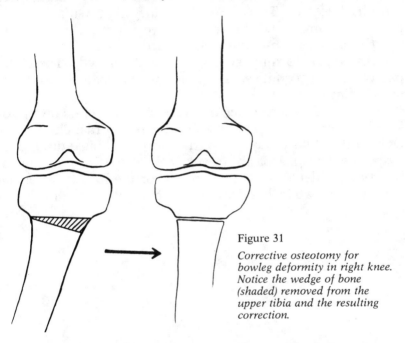

Figure 31

Corrective osteotomy for bowleg deformity in right knee. Notice the wedge of bone (shaded) removed from the upper tibia and the resulting correction.

Rickets. Rickets due to insufficient intake of vitamin D or lack of exposure to the sun is rare in this country. But rickets can also occur in children with a certain kidney disease in which the body is unable to make use of the vitamin D that has been ingested. Since bone growth is dependent on vitamin D, bone deformities including bowlegs and knock-knees may develop. The treatment is directed toward the kidney problem, since that is the underlying cause of the deformity.

Unilateral varus or valgus. Here the deformity occurs only in one knee. It is due to trauma (injury), infection, or bone tumor involving the growth plate. If the medial (inner) portion of the growth plate is involved, bowing occurs. If the lateral (outer) portion of the growth plate is involved, knock-knee is the result.

In summary, the vast majority of bowlegs and knock-knees are physiological. This means that they stay within certain prescribed limits and, in time, resolve completely. No treatment other than observation is needed. However, in rare instances, the deformity gets worse with growth. These are pathological deformities with rather distinct features, and they need definitive treatment.

Should X rays be taken of young children with bowlegs or knock-knees? The answer, in an otherwise normal child, is *no*. Only in the child where one of the aforementioned diseases is suspected because of the severity of the deformity should X rays be ordered. As long as the IC or the IM measurement stays within two inches, I would strongly advise against X ray studies.

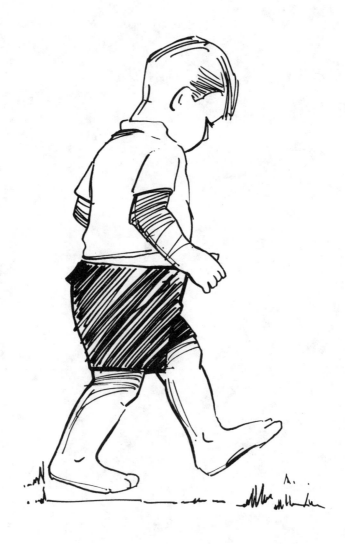

Chapter 5
Walking Woes

The textbook description of the child who walks with support around furniture at nine months of age, and who starts to toddle independently by twelve to fourteen months is just that—a textbook description. No two children are the same developmentally. Some start walking independently by the age of nine months. Others don't even try until they are fourteen to sixteen months, which could be quite worrisome to parents.

There are valid reasons for worry, for delayed walking could be due to a host of neurological and muscular problems, some of which are quite serious. It is not the purpose of this book to go into the causes of delayed walking, which is a diagnostic challenge even for the experienced physician. However, I cannot overemphasize the importance of a pediatric checkup around the child's first birthday. Many developmental milestones are reached around this age, and it is only prudent to have a medical doctor evalute the child at this juncture of his life. If he is still not walking at one, perhaps there is a good reason for it, and the pediatrician can explain that to you. If no cogent reason is found, your anxiety may be put to rest.

Toe-Walking

When the child starts to walk around fourteen months of age, his gait is initially clumsy and broad based. He tries with every step to maintain his balance while progressing. As he thrusts his foot forward, he is still learning how hard and how fast he should swing that leg, and how big a step he can take without losing his balance. He is learning by trial and error, but with each step he takes, he is learning. Moreover, until the brain learns to give the proper commands to the muscles, his movements tend to be jerky and unsteady. One of the largest muscles in his legs, the gastrocnemius muscle in the calf, tends to over pull while the child walks at this stage. Hence it is not uncommon for him to walk on tiptoes.

After about two to three months of walking, his gait becomes more steady and confident. He learns to relax and his muscles execute the commands from the brain more smoothly. His gastrocnemius muscle also learns to relax at the right time, allowing the foot to be more plantigrade, meaning the foot is now flat on the ground rather than on tiptoe.

Some children, however, continue to walk on their toes even after many months of walking. This is a fairly common problem which causes parental concern. There are three main reasons for this, each one quite common.

The first cause is heel cord tightness due to cerebral palsy and spasticity of the muscles. Cerebral palsy is a condition due to injury to the brain during or around childbirth, most often due to temporary lack of oxygen to the brain (anoxia). As a result, certain groups of muscles tighten and become spastic. One of the muscles that tightens is the gastrocnemius muscle in the calf. It is not uncommon for children with cerebral palsy to have gastrocnemius tightness alone, although other muscles are also frequently involved.

The second reason why some children persistently walk on their toes is that their heel cords are congenitally tight. They were born that way. Careful examination will not reveal any evidence of other muscle involvement, and there is no history of pregnancy or birth problems. These children form a distinct group of tight tendo-Achilles of unknown origin (idiopathic). For these children the treatment is heel cord stretching exercises, taught by the physician or physical therapist, and carried out regularly by the parents at home. If, in spite of intensive stretching exercises for three months, the gait is not improved, serial casting, bracing or even surgery may be indicated. The details of treatment should be discussed with your physician.

The third cause of persistent toe-walking is habitual toe-walking. In such a child, examination shows that the gastrocnemius and Achilles tendon are not tight. With the child lying down, his foot could be dorsiflexed to 20 degrees beyond the neutral position with ease, indicating that the Achilles tendons are of normal length. (See figure 23.) Yet as soon as he walks, his heels go up and he toe-walks.

Nagging never helps! In fact, like most childhood habits, some tend to get worse with nagging. For such a child, I would recommend gentle encouragement to plantigrade walking in the form of play ("Let's walk on our heels!") or by positive reinforcement and reward for walking right. If by the age of two years, the child has not improved, the use of plastic braces (called AFO's) to keep the ankles in the neutral position often helps to break the habit. The child may need to wear the braces about three months, the average time it takes to break the habit.

Limping and Waddling

Another common gait problem is dragging one leg while walking. This is the child who limps ever since he started to walk, in contrast to the child who has been walking normally for a while and then develops a limp. (This latter case will be discussed later.)

The child who has dragged one leg behind him ever since he started to walk may even have been dragging that same leg while he was crawling. Moreover, when he walks, he tends to swing one arm in the usual reciprocating manner, but not the other arm. Add to these observations a history of problems during pregnancy or at birth and you have a child with *hemiparetic gait.* Hemiparesis means weakness on one side of the body, usually due to brain damage at or around birth, affecting the motor area of the brain that controls the muscles of that side of the body.

Another condition that can cause a child to limp is congenital hip dislocation that had not been discovered until now.

The implications of this are serious because treatment is difficult at this age. Thanks to the vigilance of pediatricians everywhere, who routinely check hips at birth, congenital dislocation of the hip is seldom missed. However, if the condition is missed, it tends to remain undiscovered until the child starts to walk, and the hips are tested in the weight-bearing position for the first time. If one hip is dislocated, the child will drag that leg as he walks. If both hips are dislocated, the child waddles like a duck—the so-called *waddling gait*. Incidentally, a waddling gait does not necessarily mean hip dislocation. When the muscles around the hips are weak, as in muscular dystrophy, the child also waddles, even though the hips are perfectly in place.

Gait analysis is a rather complicated job, one not easily handled by a lay person. My advice to parents of young children who persistently limp or "walk funny" is to have them checked by their pediatrician, who can then make the necessary referrals when appropriate.

Refusal to Walk

It is always alarming to any parent when her hitherto healthy, active preschool child, without any apparent injury, suddenly refuses to walk. The child could either refuse to put weight on one leg, or he could do minimal walking, favoring one leg. He may even walk on his knees rather than his feet. When such a situation occurs, the parent usually imagines the worst and rushes the child to the doctor without so much as a cursory glance at the child.

Parents should do some initial evaluation at home. The following checklist will show you how.

1. *Look* at the child. Does he look sick? Does he have a fever? Then look at his legs, especially the one he is favoring. Undress the child completely and look systematically. Do not flit around. Look first at the groins, then the thighs, the knees, legs, ankles, and feet. Look for redness, swelling, bruising, or deformity. Use the other leg for comparison. Look at the foot for a buried splinter, a stone bruise in his heel, or an ingrown toenail.

2. *Feel* the whole leg, again systematically from the groin down to the foot. Is there any area that is painful to touch?

3. *Move* the joints of the whole lower extremity: the hip, knee, and ankle. Does the child dislike movement in any of these joints? Is there any stiffness? Again, use the other leg as a comparison.

If the answer to any of the questions in the checklist is affirmative, consult a doctor.

Another common yet alarming problem is the preschool child who wakes up in the middle of the night, screaming in pain. The mother may give the child an aspirin and lots of hugs and kisses; soon he falls back to sleep. The next morning he is just fine. But the following night, the whole process will happen again, and again, and again. Mother looks for any telltale signs of injury, but she finds nothing of note. When the child is not having these "attacks," he is perfectly well, playing and tumbling like any other kid on the block.

The doctor presented with a problem like this goes through a thinking process as follows:

1. Is it trauma? He looks for signs of injury and may order an X ray to determine if there is any fracture.

2. Is it infection? The child usually looks sick, has a fever, as well as redness and swelling and pain in the infected part of the body.

3. Is it a tumor? Tumors, whether benign or cancerous, are rare in children's leg bones, but an X ray often settles the question immediately.

4. Is it inflammation? Juvenile rheumatoid arthritis is rare, but it can be progressive and crippling. Blood tests may be helpful in diagnosing this condition. Kohler's disease is due to loss of blood supply to the navicular bone of the foot, causing pain in the region of the instep. This occurs in children between the ages of three and eight years of age. Rest and use of arch supports relieve the pain, and symptoms usually improve over a period of nine to twelve months. X rays will diagnose this condition quite easily.

This is by no means an exhaustive list of things that can be wrong when a child suddenly refuses to walk, or suddenly screams in pain with no apparent injury. However, any parent

can do a reasonable evaluation of her child at home before
deciding on the next course of action. Not all cases are medical
emergencies, and if a thorough check at home reveals no
significant finding, it is quite safe to observe the child at home
for a few days. In a vast majority of cases, all symtoms disappear by the third day, and no medical consultation is necessary. However, if the problem still persists for a fourth day,
seek professional advice.

Growing Pains

It is common for children without any apparent injury to
have sudden severe complaints like those just described and
just as suddenly have them disappear completely. What's the
reason for this? Many people—lay and professional—blame it
on growing pains.

"Growing pains," in my opinion, are a myth. They are a
convenient way to explain something for which we have no apparent explanation. It gives the impression that growing is
painful. I have to admit that growing up can be painful emo-
tionally, but normal physical growth should not cause pain to
the child's body.

When you look at a child at play, whether tumbling on the
grass or swinging from the tree, don't you wonder how the
child can avoid injury? He can jump from three times his
height and suffer no apparent injury. (An adult doing the same
would probably break his neck—or at least his leg!)

I venture to say that, more than likely, the child *has*
sprained some ligaments or bruised a muscle in the scuffle. Because of his high threshold to pain and the motivation to continue playing, he does not feel the pain. Afterwards, however,
he may realize that his ankle hurts. Or he may only complain of
pain after he has gone to bed, when he is relaxed and his mind
is free to give attention to the painful stimulus coming from his
injured ankle. As long as he is awake, his muscles are contract-
ing and "splinting" the injured ankle or knee, minimizing
movement and pain. But when he is asleep, the muscles relax;
with the injured knee or ankle "unsplinted," he will experience
sudden pain when he turns over in his sleep. Such pain goes
away after a few days, attesting to the rapid healing of youth.

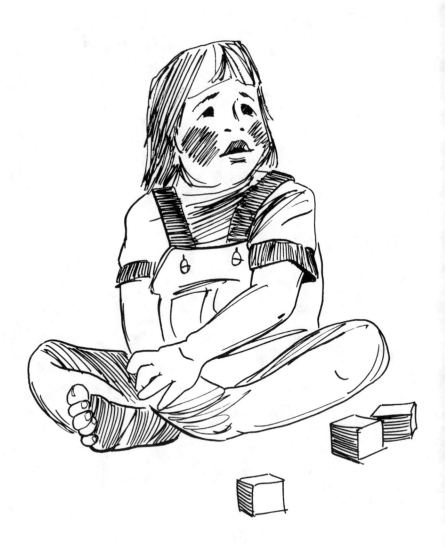

Chapter 6
Bunions and Curly Toes

A frequently encountered problem in infants and children is crooked toes. To understand this problem, look briefly at the anatomy of the toe.

The toe is made up of a series of articulated little bones called phalanges, joined at their bases to the foot. The joint between the foot (metatarsal bone) and the toe is the metatarso-phalangeal joint (**MP** joint). The joints between the three phalanges of the toe are the proximal and distal interphalangeal joints.

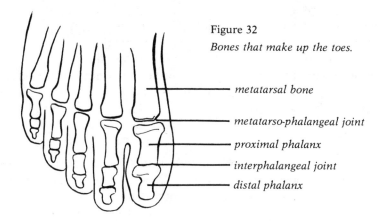

Figure 32
Bones that make up the toes.

metatarsal bone

metatarso-phalangeal joint

proximal phalanx

interphalangeal joint

distal phalanx

Hammertoe

This deformity occurs at the proximal interphalangeal joint (PIP joint). If present at birth, it is probably due to genetic factors, as it tends to run in families. If the deformity occurs as the child grows older, it is probably due to faulty shoes. Shoes that are too small or narrow can cause bunions and hammertoes.

In the infant and young child, passive stretching exercises by the parents at home followed by strapping with adhesive tape may be helpful, though maybe not curative. As chapter 7 will explain, the infant and young child should not be in shoes all day. Feet and toes need a chance to stretch and develop normally. As the child grows older and needs to be in shoes for longer periods of time, parents should take care to select shoes that have an adequate toe box so that the hammertoe deformity will not be made worse.

In the older child or adolescent, if the deformity continues to be mild, it is usually asymptomatic and is best left alone. However, if the deformity is severe and causes pain, surgical excision of the proximal interphalangeal joint may be necessary.

Mallet Toe

This deformity occurs at the distal interphalangeal joint (DIP joint) so that only the tip of the toe is crooked. (See figure.) In the infant or young child, it is usually not painful, and stretching exercises and adhesive tape strapping may be helpful. In the older child, this deformity may cause development of a painful corn at the tip of the toe. Shaving of the corn and appropriate padding would relieve the pain. In the extreme case, correction of the deformity by surgical fusion of the DIP joint may be necessary.

Claw Toe

Claw toe is a relatively rare condition, but when present, it involves all the joints of the toe: hyperextension deformity at the MP joint and flexion deformity at both the PIP and DIP joints. (See figure.) Usually all the toes are involved.

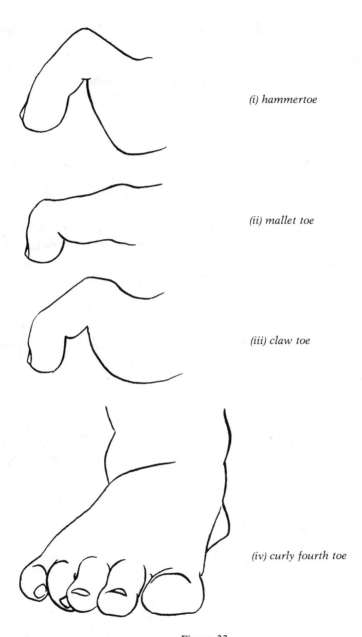

(i) hammertoe

(ii) mallet toe

(iii) claw toe

(iv) curly fourth toe

Figure 33

Claw toe is associated with foot deformities or neuro-logical or muscular problems like spina bifida. It is disabling, not because of the clawing, but because of the primary disease which causes severe problems in the legs. The treatment of claw toe is only part of the overall management of the under-lying primary disease and foot deformities.

Congenital Curly Toe

This is a fairly common problem that tends to run in fam-ilies. It usually affects the fourth or fifth toes and often involves both feet. The affected toes are flexed downward and twisted underneath the adjacent toes. In infancy and childhood, the condition is not symptomatic and no treatment is needed. Some doctors may advise strapping. This is difficult to do on an infant, and the results are uncertain. In the rare case where the deformity is very severe, surgical release of the toe tendons may correct the deformity.

Children with curly toes who have been followed into adulthood continue to have no problems with their toes. This can be ascertained by asking the parents of children with curly toes. These parents often have the same deformity in their toes, but with no symptoms.

Extra Toes

Some children are born with extra toes (polydactyly). If the duplication is one of the middle toes, no treatment is indicated.

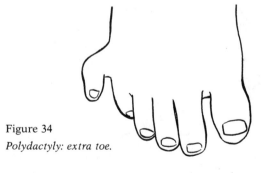

Figure 34
Polydactyly: extra toe.

However, if the duplication occurs in the big or little toe and the extra toe sticks out prominently, it should be excised before the age of one to facilitate wearing shoes.

Webbed Toes

Unlike webbing of fingers where treatment is invariably needed for proper individual finger function, webbing of toes (syndactyly) does not require surgical separation for functional or cosmetic reasons.

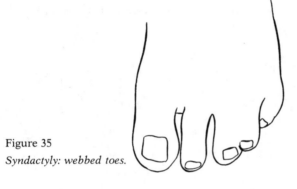

Figure 35
Syndactyly: webbed toes.

Bunions

In bunion deformity (hallux valgus) the great toe is deviated away from the midline at the metatarso-phalangeal

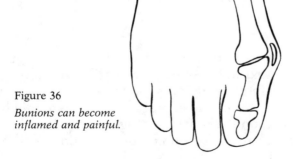

Figure 36

Bunions can become inflamed and painful.

joint (MP joint). As the deformity progresses, the normal bunion or prominence at this joint is irritated by constant pressure from the shoe; it becomes red, inflamed, and painful.

Here are the main causes of this problem:

1. Untreated metatarsus adductus where the forefoot deviates inward, or hallux varus where the big toe deviates inward. These two conditions are often present at the same time. With shoe wear (even good shoes), the great toe is pushed outward; over a period of years the typical bunion deformity develops.

2. Pointed, stylized shoes squeeze the toes because there is not enough room in the toe box area to accommodate them. This is the best-documented cause of bunions as the following diagram illustrates.

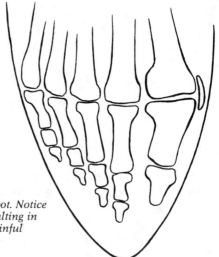

Figure 37

Effect of pointed shoe on the foot. Notice how the toes are squashed, resulting in bunions at the great toe and painful callosities at the little toe.

Progressive compression of the big toe causes bunion deformity, and, at the same time, the little toe develops a callus. Both are painful. Symptoms can arise at any age. Although the deformity may not cause problems until late middle age, it is not uncommon to see it in teenagers as well.

The treatment for bunion depends on the severity of the condition. If the deformity is mild, wearing shoes with a roomy toe box will prevent the deformity from getting worse. If the deformity is severe and painful, surgical correction may be required. However, prevention is always much better than cure; hence the reason for the next chapter.

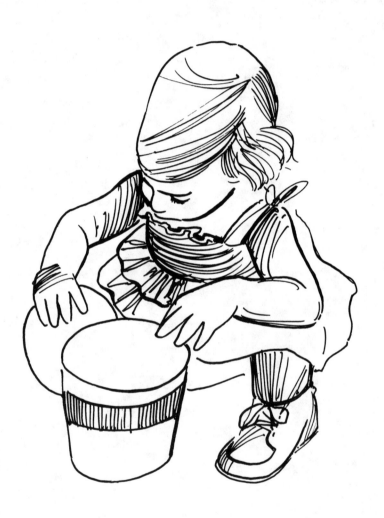

Chapter 7
Selecting Shoes for Children

Shoes are a necessary evil. If the whole world were all soft earth covered with a carpet of grass and leaves, there would be no need for shoes. However, since the modern-day world in which we live is, in large part, paved with hard, unforgiving concrete and littered with sharp remnants of glass and the like, the foot needs protection from injury.

Although the adult shoe has changed from being a protective covering to becoming a status symbol, the child's shoe has remained in its basic role—protecting the foot from the hazards of the outside world.

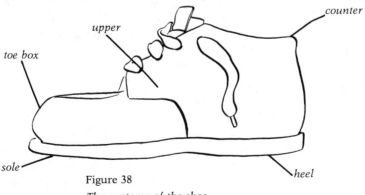

Figure 38
The anatomy of the shoe.

However, there is a great deal of confusion regarding the choice of appropriate shoes for children with normal feet. A recent survey of professionals who give advice on children's feet (pediatricians, orthopedic surgeons, pediatric orthopedists, podiatrists) revealed wide divergence of opinion regarding shoes and footwear in both normal and problem feet. Not only is there difference in opinion between each group of practitioners, but marked differences occur among members of the same group. Of all the practitioners surveyed, 15 percent thought that, in general, high-topped "orthopedic" shoes contributed to normal foot development; 85 percent disagreed. In the same survey, 44 percent recommended soft shoes for infants, 32 percent recommended high-topped shoes, and 24 percent, tennis shoes.

What is a parent to do? I feel that the only rational approach to the subject is to examine some "traditional" ideas in the light of recent studies and experience and determine if they should be upheld or discarded.

1. "Shoes are necessary to promote foot development." In other words, normal children's feet need support, otherwise they will become flat.

Recent studies seem to contradict this. Feet deformities, like bunions and hammertoes, are very rare among primitive people who wear no shoes, in contrast to advanced cultures, where such deformities are commonly seen. A study in England revealed that among children two to four years of age, 80 percent of those who constantly wore shoes had deflection of the terminal phalanx of the great toe, and 30 percent had incurving of the fourth and fifth toes. These deformities were not found in children who had not worn shoes.

Perhaps the most conclusive study was the one that compared foot forms among the non-shoe and the shoe-wearing Chinese population in Hong Kong. The incidence of hallux valgus, hallux rigidus, incurved fifth toe, hammertoe, and a host of other foot and toe deformities was much higher in the shoe-wearing population. The study concluded that the foot in its natural, unrestricted form is mobile and flexible and free of the structural problems so often encountered in the shoe-wearing population.

These observations lead one to conclude that shoes are not necessary for normal foot development. A normal foot does not need shoe support. In fact, heavy shoes, unless prescribed for a specific problem, do more harm than good.

2. "High-top shoes are necessary to support the ankle as the child takes his first steps."

This myth is often perpetrated by well-meaning but misinformed relatives. Studies have shown that when a child is old enough and strong enough to stand up and walk, he will have ankles strong enough to support his body. If he is not ready to walk, propping him up with high-top shoes is not only ineffective, but probably detrimental to his feet.

Parents may still want to put their toddler in high-top shoes. They should use them to prevent the child from kicking off his shoes rather than in the mistaken belief that somehow the shoes support his ankles.

3. "Sneakers, if worn for more than a couple of hours a day, are bad for children."

This is a widely held belief among lay people as well as professionals. There is absolutely no evidence that normal feet develop into flatfeet if tennis shoes rather than high-top or leather shoes are used.

Dr. E. Bleck of Stanford University followed forty children with normal feet over a period of ten years. These children wore sneakers and nothing else. He found no tendency at all toward flatfeet.

Granted, not all sneakers are created equal. But a good pair of sneakers should not cause any foot problems if used appropriately.

4. "A high arch is important for normal foot function."

Parents frequently come into the office complaining that their child's feet are flat. A close examination indicates that, although the feet have low arches, they are by no means flat. (See chapter 3.) Children with apparent flatfeet (or low arches), when followed over long periods of time, do not develop functional problems.

A classic study done by a famous orthopedic surgeon in Toronto some years ago on Canadian army recruits revealed that 22 percent of the recruits had the appearance of flatfeet, but were actually low arches. They were all asymptomatic with no problems whatsoever.

5. "Shoe salesmen are competent to diagnose foot problems and advise remedial shoe wear for children."

This is totally erroneous. Most shoe salesmen are well intentioned and desire to sell you the most comfortable shoes they can find. But they are not trained to give advice regarding foot problems. The responsible salesman may suggest to the parent that the child's feet do not appear right and he would recommend that the child be seen by a doctor; but the salesman certainly will not suggest any kind of corrective shoes without a doctor's prescription. Remember, too, that the salesman is there to make a sale. He is there to help you choose the most appropriate pair of shoes possible, but the responsibility of selecting the proper shoes for your child lies with you, the parent.

A recent survey of parents revealed that they most often obtain information about shoes from friends, relatives, and shoe salesmen. Only a minority talk to their pediatricians about their children's shoes. An interesting finding of the study was that the parents who got advice from their physicians spent the least on shoes, while the parents who got most of their information from salesmen spent the most for shoes. Shoe salesmen tend to recommend shoes with hard soles, high tops, laces, and steel shanks. These are not only costly, they are also unnecessary and possibly harmful for some children.

I do not want you to view the shoe salesman in an adversarial position. He knows the variety of shoes he has in stock and can advise you as to what is available when you tell him the features you are looking for. The following guidelines will help you know how to select shoes for your child.

The Age for Shoes

Now that you know shoes are unnecessary for foot support and development, it is only logical to conclude that, for normal feet, shoes serve only one function: protection. In the first year of life before the child begins to walk, he does not need shoes. If the pre-walker has shoes on constantly, he is deprived of the normal sensory stimulation his feet would otherwise get from contact with the environment. Moreover, the small muscles of his feet and toes do not get much chance for exercise and tend to underdevelop.

Even the toddler does not generally need shoes when he is in the safe environs of his home or backyard. Only for going out on the street is a pair of sneakers necessary for protection.

The Price of Shoes

The price of shoes is often related to the kind of material used. Leather is the most expensive, especially if it is used for both uppers and soles. Since leather allows the feet to "breathe" in the shoes, it helps avoid sweat accumulation and skin irritation. While leather uppers are desirable, leather soles are not necessary. Buying shoes with leather uppers and rubber or crepe soles will cut down on the price considerably.

It is not necessary to get the most durable or expensive children's shoes. The chief reason for replacing shoes is that children outgrow them. High quality, long lasting shoes are therefore an unnecessary expense.

Sneakers are much less expensive. They have cloth or canvas uppers, and, like leather, allow the feet to "breathe." The exception are running shoes with rubber bindings which tend to cause sweat accumulation if worn for long periods of time. The rubber bindings, however, make the shoes more waterproof—a distinct advantage on wet days. On the whole, sneakers that have the desired qualities that we shall discuss serve just as well as the more expensive leather shoes.

I advise a pair of good sneakers or running shoes for everyday wear for most children. Even then, they should be allowed to be without shoes for part of the day. Young children feel as much with their feet as with their hands, and sensory input is essential for brain development. Moreover, exposing the feet allows for ventilation and prevents sweat buildup and skin problems.

The Soles of Shoes

The soles of the shoes, whether leather or rubber, should be thick enough to protect, yet flexible enough for walking. It is also important to look at the bottom of the soles to determine the depth of the grooves. The deeper the grooves, the better the traction. These kinds of shoes can be used in wet weather and even wintertime with no slippage problems.

Flexibility in the sole is very important. The normal foot flexes at the metatarso-phalangeal joints, moving through a range of 30 to 40 degrees during normal walking. A good shoe should allow this. Sneakers are admirably suited in this respect. Rigid soles, unless prescribed by a physician for a specific problem, should be avoided.

The way to test flexibility is by bending the shoe upward. The sole should bend in the ball area without much effort on your part.

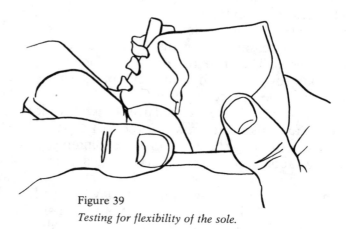

Figure 39
Testing for flexibility of the sole.

The Shoe Counter

If you look at the back of your child's feet while he is standing, you will notice that the heel cords (tendo-Achilles) deviate slightly outward away from each other as you follow them down to the heels.

A firm, substantial shoe counter is necessary to prevent the counter from becoming deformed. If it is flimsy, the slight offset of the heel cord and ankle will cause the counter to deviate inward and the hindfoot will not sit squarely on the shoe as it should.

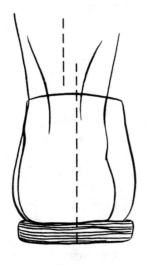

Figure 40

Right heel in shoe. The slight offset between the axis of the leg and the axis of the shoe puts stress on the shoe counter. Hence the need for a firm and substantial shoe counter.

Children tend to abuse their shoes. How many times have you seen your child run out to play while his shoes are only half on and the heel of the foot is still on the shoe counter, squashing it in the process? A flimsy shoe counter will not be able to withstand this abuse. It will lose its support very quickly.

A padded counter is also important. Run your finger along the inside of the shoe counter. Check to see if there is anything hard or irregular that could cause irritation to the back of the child's heel.

The Heels on Shoes

Children's shoes should not have heels. Heels encourage the child to walk on his toes, and this causes tightening of the heel cords. High heels should definitely be avoided. Most leather shoes have a slight heel. If worn occasionally, this does not matter. But sneakers or running shoes are ideal in this regard.

Fitting Children's Shoes

You must remember that you are looking for a pair of shoes to fit your child's feet, not vice versa. To get a good fit, both the shape and the size of the shoes should conform to his feet.

No two feet are identical in all respects. Unless shoes are custom-made, there is no such thing as the "perfect fit." For perfect fit, you not only have to get shoes of adequate overall length and width, but they also have to satisfy other considerations. The widest part of the foot may not be seated in the corresponding widest part of the shoe, even though they may be of the same width. Also, the width of the heel may not fit the heel of the shoe. However, this does not mean that one cannot find shoes that are comfortable and that generally conform to the shape and size of the foot.

Foot size increases with standing as well as with the time of day. Feet are slightly longer and wider at the end of the day. The average adult foot increases 4 percent in volume from morning to night. This translates to an increase of foot width of up to one-half inch (or two sizes) and length of up to one-eighth inch (or one-half size). While no formal study has been done in children, I believe that proportionate increases could be expected. I would therefore recommend that you shop for shoes later in the day when feet are at their largest.

Even while you are looking at the different shoes in the store, keep in mind the shape of the shoe that you should be looking for. The shape of the shoe is determined by the last, which is the model from which the shoe is made. You want a straight last, since this conforms best to the shape of your child's foot. Most shoes for preschool children are made from straight lasts. Unfortunately, due to the dictates of fashion and profitability, many lasts for older children have been flared inward. If you imagine the shoe like the foot, consisting of a back part and a forepart, the forepart is angled inward. Such a shoe would force the foot into an adducted or in-toe position, much like the metatarsus adductus discussed in chapter 2.

In addition, some shoe manufacturers have stylized the toe box, making it more pointed. This squeezes the toes together in an unnatural position and is a frequent cause of bunions and other toe deformities in children.

The way to determine flare is not by looking at the bottom of the shoes; the undercut of the shank area and the trimmings of the outsole may be deceptive. The way to determine flare is to look at the shoes from above. Visually gauge the shape of the shoe as a whole to determine if the forepart flares inward. Also determine at the same time if the toe box has been stylized and pointed.

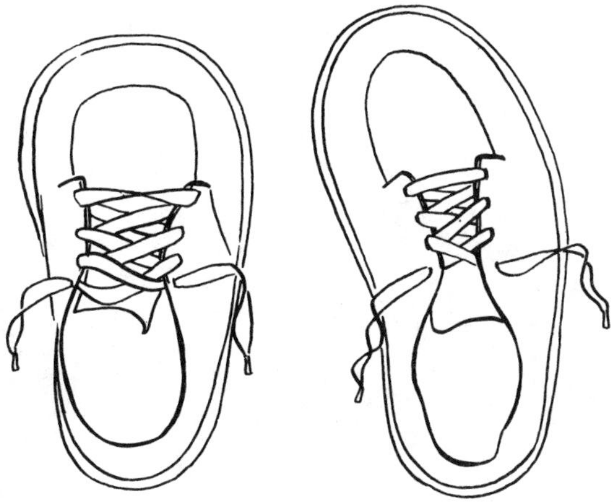

Figure 41

Visually gauge the shape of the shoe as a whole to determine if the forepart is straight (i) or flared inward (ii).

(i)   (ii)

When you have decided on a few styles which are acceptable to you on the basis of the last, you are ready for the salesman.

Always have the salesman measure your child's feet, rather than just telling him what size you think is right. When being measured, the child should be standing up and putting full weight on his feet. If there is a size difference between the feet, take the larger size.

There is nothing magical about the measurements. They are not necessarily the right size for your child. The measurements only give you a place to start. Once the shoes are on, they should be checked for adequate length and width. With the child standing, check the toe box to make sure the toes have plenty of room. You should be able to feel a thumb's space between the end of the toes and the tip of the shoe. For adequate width, check the broadest part of the foot which is at the ball of the foot. Feel the shoe. It should not be bulging out, indicating tightness, and you should be able to get a pinch of leather or canvas. With the child still standing, see if there is enough room behind his heel to insert your little finger. This ensures that the shoe has enough growing room in the back. Remember that the foot grows backward as well as forward.

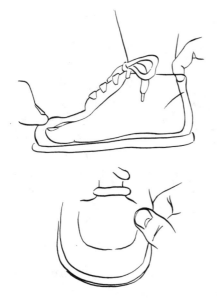

Figure 42

Shoe fitting: (1) toe box is rounded and roomy, not pointed; (2) thumb space between the ends of the toes and the tip of the shoe; (3) tip of little finger between the heel and counter at the back; (4) pinch of leather or canvas at the widest part of the shoe.

Have the child wear the shoes and walk around the store for about five minutes. Then quickly remove the shoes and examine his feet for any redness. Check especially the little toes, the widest part of the foot at the base of the great toe, and the back of the heels. Redness is an indication of pressure on these areas. Do not accept discomfort as a normal "breaking in" process. Feet could break in the process!

A child may be stoical about discomfort and not complain, even if shoes are too tight or constrictive. But if he tends to remove his shoes frequently, limps, or refuses to walk whenever he is in shoes, take note and suspect misfit. Keep in mind, too, that children's feet have a way of growing out of their shoes.

Frequency of Size Change

The most common reason for replacing children's shoes is that they have been outgrown. Some people in the shoe industry have recommended that shoe size should be changed every two months for children between the ages of two and six. While this is great for the shoe industry, it is prohibitively expensive. This recommendation is not based on any longitudinal study of children's foot growth.

Fortunately for parents, more recent studies by the medical profession have revealed that while children's foot growth is rapid, changes in shoe size need not be that frequent. Between the ages of twelve to thirty months, foot growth is explosive, and, indeed, size change should be considered every three months. However, from three to six years of age, the foot grows much less rapidly, and one needs to check for size change only once every four to six months.

Every child's growth is different, and one should not be negligent in replacing outgrown shoes. Habitual use of outgrown shoes can cause foot and toe deformities, not to mention the discomfort inflicted on the child.

Handing Down Shoes

The shoe industry frowns on handing down shoes. The feeling is that the old shoes bear the imprint of the previous owner's feet, and this may cause problems for the new owner. While this may be true in some cases, it is not the rule. Needless to say, handing down shoes should be practiced only within the family. Never wear shoes that belonged to strangers, since shoes can be a source of disease transmission.

The wise parent likes to save money whenever she can, but not at the expense of foot health. She will examine the old shoes to make sure they are in good condition before handing them down to the next child. She will *not* hand shoes down if:

1. The previous owner had feet problems like true flatfeet or metatarsus adductus.

2. The heels or soles of the shoes are unevenly worn. This usually indicates feet problems in the previous owner.

3. The counter of the shoe is deformed or badly creased from previous abuse.

4. The uppers of the shoes, especially at the toe box, have been stretched out or are bulging, indicating previous misfit. Put your hand into the shoes and feel for any grooves from excessive wear. If any are present, it is best not to reuse the shoes.

If, after carefully examining the shoes, you find them in good condition, there is no reason why you should not save yourself some unnecessary expenses.

Chapter 8
Here's to Happy Feet!

Having come to the last chapter of this book, you have begun to understand a little about your child's legs and feet. You also realize how their appearance evolves from birth through early childhood. In-toeing, out-toeing, flatfeet, bowlegs, knock-knees, and toe-walking, if within prescribed limits, are now less worrisome to you. You now know that they will, in time, pass away. You also have learned how to select shoes for your child's feet, which will stand him in good stead for the future.

This book has not been written so that you can self-diagnose and self-treat your child. In spite of the knowledge you have, you will want to consult with a professional on some occasions. Do you then go to your pediatrician, family doctor, orthopedic surgeon, or pediatric orthopedist? As the intent of this book is not to elevate one group of doctors over another, my answer to this frequently asked question is to seek out someone who has experience and interest in treating children's leg and feet problems.

For most parents, the first call should be to your pediatrician or family doctor. Explain to him your concerns. In many cases, his advice is all you need. But after talking to him, if you still have some concern that you feel has not been addressed, let him know. He will be happy to refer you for a second opinion. (Contrary to what you think, most doctors do not get offended if you would like a second opinion. They are concerned that the child gets the best treatment that is available.) Go ahead with another opinion if you so desire, but let your pediatrician or family doctor know with whom you intend to consult. This makes for better communication between doctors, with your child as the ultimate benefactor of this dialogue.

Children's feet are hardy things and are made to last for life. If some thought and care are given to them while they are young, those feet should give them many, many years of happy walking.

Here's to happy feet!

Appendix

Anatomy of the Foot

The leg bones (tibia and fibula) articulate with the foot at the ankle joint. The foot is made up of twenty-six bones, articulating at multiple joints in a complex relationship. These bones are joined together by ligaments, which give them support, and by muscles and tendons, which give the joints mobility.

The best way to understand the foot in a functional way is to divide the foot into two sections: the hindfoot and the forefoot.

The hindfoot consists of two fairly big bones: the talus and the calcaneus. The top surface of the talus articulates with the tibia and fibula at the ankle joint, while the lower surface of the talus articulates with the calcaneus at the subtalar joint. Together, the talus and the calcaneus articulate with the forefoot at the midtarsal joint.

The forefoot consists of the navicular and cuboid bones, which articulate with the talus and calcaneus of the hindfoot at the midtarsal joint, as well as the cuneiform bones, and the metatarsal and phalangeal bones of each of the five digits.

The ankle joint is a hinge joint, and, like the hinge of a door, moves in one axis only. It allows the foot as a whole to

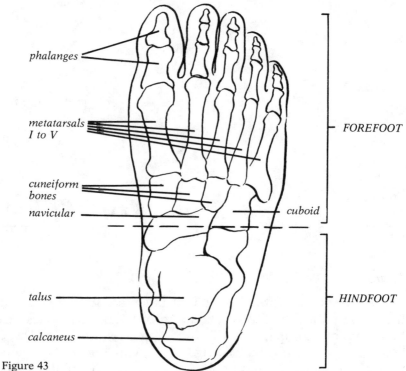

Figure 43

The hindfoot consists of the talus and calcaneus. The forefoot consists of all other bones of the foot.

Figure 44

Bones of the foot showing the sites of the three major joints of the foot where most of the motion occurs.

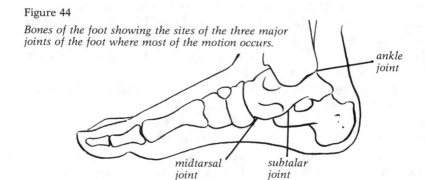

flex upward (called dorsiflexion) or downward (called plantar-flexion).

The subtalar joint is also a hinge joint, but it moves in an axis perpendicular to the ankle joint, allowing you to bring your foot inward toward the midline (called inversion) or outward away from the midline (called eversion).

The midtarsal joint allows the forefoot to turn in relative to the hindfoot (called adduction) or turn out (called abduction).

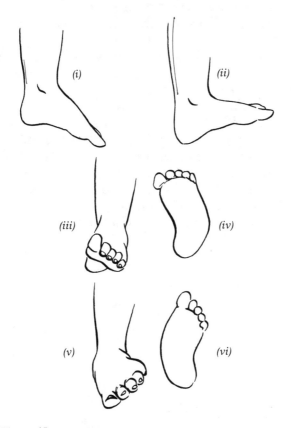

Figure 45

The ankle joint allows for plantarflexion (i) or dorsiflexion (ii).
The subtalar joint allows for inversion (iii) or eversion (v).
The midtarsal joint allows for adduction (iv) or abduction (vi).
Inversion (iii) and adduction (iv) tend to occur together.
Eversion (v) and abduction (vi) tend to occur together.

Anatomical Basis of Common Foot Deformities

The normal foot can be held voluntarily in the so-called neutral position, with the foot perpendicular to the leg, and held in a straight forward position.

If the foot is fixed in the plantarflexed position at the ankle, the deformity is called an equinus position. This occurs when the tendo-Achilles (heel cords) are tight, and the child will toe-walk. If the foot is fixed in the dorsiflexed position, it is called a calcaneus deformity. This occurs commonly at birth as postural calcaneo-valgus, which tends to improve spontaneously with time. A much rarer, but more serious calcaneus deformity, occurs in children with spina bifida and other neurological conditions. Such children often have significant problems in other parts of the body as well.

If the subtalar joint is fixed in the inverted position, it is called a varus deformity. This, along with equinus, is the typical deformity of congenital clubfoot. If the subtalar joint is fixed in the everted position, the deformity is called a valgus deformity, and occurs in children with severe flatfeet.

If the midtarsal joint is held in the adducted position, the typical deformity is called metatarsus adductus, a very common cause of in-toeing in young children.

Index